DISCOURSES

ON THE

SOBER LIFE

Louis Cornaro lived to be 102 in the fifteenth & sixteenth centuries. He was told at the age of 40 he didn't have long to live. He reformed his diet and mode of living and reached an age quite unusual for his era. First Discourse: On a temperate & healthful life; Second Discourse: Showing the surest method of correcting an infirm constitution; Third Discourse: The method of enjoying complete happiness in old age; Fourth Discourse: An exhortation to a sober & regular life, in order to attain old age.

INTRODUCTION BY

HEREWARD CARRINGTON & HERBERT M. SHELTON

Luigi Cornaro

ISBN 1-56459-655-9

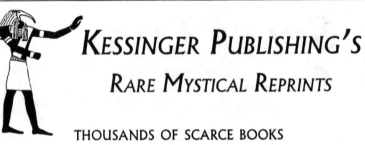
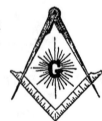

The most remarkable instance of the efficacy of temperance toward the procuring of long life, is what we meet with in a little book published by Luigi Cornaro, the Venetian; which I the rather mention, because it is of undoubted credit, as the late Venetian ambassador, who was of the same family, attested more than once in conversation, when he resided in England. Cornaro, who was the author of the little "Treatise" I am mentioning, was of an infirm constitution, till about forty, when, by obstinately persisting in an exact course of temperance, he recovered a perfect state of health; insomuch that at fourscore he published his book, which has been translated into English under the title "A Sure and Certain Method of Attaining a Long and Healthy Life." He lived to give a third or fourth edition of it; and, after having passed his hundredth year, died without pain or agony, and like one who falls asleep. The "Treatise" I mention has been taken notice of by several eminent authors, and is written with such a spirit of cheerfulness, religion and good sense, as are the natural concomitants of temperance and sobriety. The mixture of the old man in it is rather a recommendation than a discredit to it.—JOSEPH ADDISON, in "The Spectator."

INTRODUCTION

By Hereward Carrington

This famous work, by Louis Cornaro, *The Temperate Life*, (sometimes titled, *How to Live 100 Years*), has been translated into many different languages. Yet it is hardly known to anyone today. But it is one of the greatest books on Hygiene ever written, and Health Research is certainly to be congratulated in having made this reprint of it, thereby bringing it before the reading public.

Cornaro was a Venetian nobleman, four of his ancestors having been Doges of the "Serene Republic." He was born in 1464, and lived to the age of 102, dying in 1566. Like the majority of young gallants of his day, Louis Cornaro lived a reckless and dissipated life, the result being that he completely broke-down, at the age of forty, and was given-up by his physicians to die. He was indeed a physical wreck!

Taking matters into his own hands, however, Cornaro decided to reform his life, and see what the results would be. He simplified his diet and cut down on the quantity of food to the barest minimum. Within a few days he began to see the difference, and at the end of a year found himself completely restored to health. Seeing this, he continued this simple and abstemious life for the rest of his life. He limited himself to twelve ounces of solid food daily - and fourteen ounces of wine. (If the modern Hygienist should raise his eye-brows at this, he should remember that wine, in the Latin countries, is very light, and is drunk by them at meals, just as we drink water. It is taken as a matter-of-course. Fourteen ounces is a comparatively small amount.)

Cornaro's book, "La Vita Sobria," consists of four "Discourses," the first being written at the age of eighty-three, the second at eighty-six, the third at ninety-one, and the fourth at ninety-five. To the end of his life Cornaro continued to lead an active and useful existence, devoting much of his time and energy to the spreading of these doctrines and in attempts to spread the knowledge of dietetic reform. It is safe to say that, since his work was published, many thousands have regained health and prolonged their lives by reason of his teachings.

While these are fully set forth in the treatise which follows, I can-not refrain from quoting a few brief passages, which illustrate how "modern" many of his views were, and how true a *"Hygienist"* he really was. Take the following sentences, for example:

". . . And there is no doubt that if the one so advised were to act accordingly, he would avoid all sickness in the future; because a well-regulated life removes the *causes* of disease. Thus, for the remainder of his days, he would have no further need either of doctors or of medicines."

"Should he, when ill, continue to eat the same amount as when in health, he would surely die; while, were he to eat more, he would die all the sooner. For his natural powers, already oppressed with sickness, would thereby be burdened beyond endurance, having had forced upon them a quantity of food greater than they could support under the circumstances. A reduced quantity, is, in my opinion, all that is required to sustain the individual.''

And again:

''. . . . I accustomed myself to the habit of never fully satisfying my appetite, either with eating or drinking - always leaving the table when able to take more. In this I acted according to the Proverb: Not to satiate one's self with food is the science of health.''

How in accordance with our modern teachings!

Various editions of Cornaro's work have appeared in English translations. One of the earliest of these, editions, it seems, was issued in 1842, under the editorial supervision of Dr. John Burdell: another edition, undated, was published by the Crowell Company, and still another by the Health Culture Co., of New York in 1916. Meanwhile a little-known edition was issued in 1903, by William F. Butler, of Milwaukee. The latest to see the light of day is an English version, published in 1951, by the ''Health for All Publishing Company.''

Addison, writing in ''The Spectator,'' (October 13, 1711), paid a glowing tribute to Cornaro; and so did Lord Bacon, in his ''History of Life and Death.'' and Sir William Temple, in his ''Health and Long Life,'' (16th cent.), while on August 10, 1817, Bartholomeo Gamba, - - a noted author in his day, - - delivered an address before the Royal Academy of

Fine Arts of Venice, which consisted of a Eulogy of Louis Cornaro. Cornaro's sumptuous palace still stands in Padua, and may be visited by any tourist who is sufficiently interested to do so. Cornaro was the Administrator of the Bishopric of Padua for many years, under Cardinal Pisani. It is said that, in Italy, his work is still considered one of the "classics."

It is evident, therefore, that Cornaro's influence has been long and enduring, and it is high time that modern health reformers should realize this and estimate him at his true worth. No one in the Middle Ages exerted so great an influence.

Cornaro emphasizes several points in his Treatise which are perhaps too often overlooked by the modern health enthusiast. He points out, first of all, that mere prolongation of life is in itself useless unless that life is healthy and contented. A long life full of disease and misery is worse than no life at all. The object of health should be, rather, to enable us to forget the body, and to carry on our interests and life-activities without impediment or interference, because of sickness or debility, thus permitting the free and full use of our faculties and talents. In short, we should DO something with our lives, besides merely living them; and the object of health is to insure this possibility, making a useful and constructive life possible. Health, then, is merely a means to an end, rather than an end in itself. (But, of course, until health is attained, it must be our primary object to attain it!)

This point-of-view was endorsed and indeed emphasized by both Bacon and Temple, the latter writing:

"The two great blessings of life are, in my opinion, health and good humor; and none contribute more to one another. Without health, all will allow life to be but a burden; and the several conditions of fortune to be all wearisome, dull, or disagreeable, without good humor . . . . The vigor of the mind decays with that of the body, and not only humor and invention, but even judgment and resolution, change and languish with ill-constitution of body and of health . . .

"That which I call temperance is a regular and simple diet, limited by every man's experience of his own easy digestion, and thereby proportioning, as near as well as can be, the daily repairs to the daily, decays of our wasting bodies . . .

"In the course of common life, a man must either often exercise, or rest, or take physic, or be sick; and the choice seems left to everyone as he likes. The first two are the best methods and means of preserving health . . . 'Tis true, physicians must be in danger of losing their credit with the vulgar if they should often tell a patient he has no need of physic, and prescribe only rules of diet or common use; most people would think they had lost their fee. But the first excellence of a physician's skill and care is discovered by resolving whether it be best in the case to administer any physic or none - - to trust to nature or to art; and the next, to give such prescriptions as, if they do no good, may be sure to do no harm."

Bacon, again, writes in much the same strain. He says:

"To preserve long life, the body of man must be considered . . . Age is nothing of itself, being only the measure of time . . . . A pythagorian diet according to strict rules, and always exactly equal - as that of Cornaro - seemeth to be very effectual for long life. If there were anything eminent in the Spartans, that was to be imputed to the parsimony of their diet . . . Certainly this is without all question: diet, well ordered, bears the greatest part in the prolongation of life . . .

"Hope is the most beneficial of all the affections, and doth much for the prolongation of life, if it be not too often frustrated, but entertaineth the fancy with an expectation of good; therefore they which fix and propound to themselves some end - as the mark and scope of their life - and continually and by degrees go forward in the same, are, for the most part, long-lived."

Yet there are some who contend that "psychosomatic medicine" and the teachings of "new thought" and "applied psychology" are really new!

Cornaro was indeed a pioneer, and if there are some today who may think that there is nothing essentially novel in what he said, we must remember that, in his day, science, as we understand it, was almost an unknown factor; physiology had hardly been born

14

and psychology undreamed of. Our knowledge of fasting, dietetics, food combinations, organic foods, etc., all came into being almost within the memory of men yet living - though many of the essentials were propounded by the great health reformers of the last century. (See *The Fasting Story* and *The History of Natural Hygiene*, both published by Health Research). Today we have a wealth of material to draw upon, as well as vast experience and the means of disseminating this knowledge. But when Cornaro wrote, none of this was in being. It is all the more remarkable, therefore, that he was enabled to write as he did, for the *whys* and *hows* of this method were not discovered until centuries later!

Cornaro himself, it seems, never actually fasted - - merely reducing the quantity of food which he ate to an absolute minimum. The consequence was that it took him nearly a year to regain full health, whereas he could probably have achieved the same result within a month, had he taken more drastic measures. However, he did ultimately attain a state of excellent health, and for the ensuing sixty-odd years he maintained it by reason of his abstemious life. There is no reason why anyone could not do likewise!

Indeed, there is every reason why a man today should not do even better, for the things which constituted the basis of Cornaro's diet would be spurned by the modern Hygienist. Bread, eggs and the lighter meats were his staple foods, and practically no mention is made anywhere of fruits, salads, etc., which play so important a role in the reformed diet of today. Many of these were doubtless unknown and unprocurable when he lived, so that we should profit by the quality of the food we eat no less than by the quantity. But the mere fact that Cornaro regained and maintained his health, on his diet, shows us how important a factor the restriction of quantity is, and indicates that this is, in all probability, the most important single factor in the preservation of health and longevity . . . .

Cornaro's book was one of the first I read when I began my reading on *Natural Hygiene*, and the fact that I am writing this Introduction to the book now is something of a thrill. I presume that *Health Research* asked me to write this prefactory material because they know that I am now long past seventy myself, and am one of the few surviving early health reformers . . . I suppose I am one of the few people living today who can truthfully say that he has never had a serious illness in his life, and never been inside a hospital, save as a visitor! But there is no reason why practically everyone could not say the same thing; the maintenance of health is such an easy matter that it seems almost odd that anyone should become ill! And if anyone asks how this desirable condition is to be brought about, one cannot do better than refer him to Cornaro's book, - - supplementing this by up-to-date advice and information on dietetics and general hygiene. There can be no

16

doubt that a vital, healthy human race would result
in consequence, - - instead of the miserable and dis-
ease-ridden humanity that we see everywhere about
us! Cornaro's great work should prove an important
factor in achieving this desirable result. It is with
this hope that the book is sent-forth on its mission!

Introduction

By Herbert M. Shelton

In 1833 an edition of Cornaro's *Discourses on a Sober and Temperate Life* was published in New York with introduction and notes by Sylvester Graham. Mr. Graham edited and corrected the edition and it was presented to the reading public of that day in the hope, a not vain one, that it would result in the people becoming more sober and temperate in their ways of life. Many read the book with understanding and followed its precepts with profit. A number of editions of this renowned book have been published since that time and I believe it safe to say that few books of its kind have ever exerted a wide and more wholesome influence.

In his introduction Graham demolished the opinion then held and still held by the great majority of people who give thought to the subject at all, that, "every man can ascertain, by his own *experience*, what is best for him, and how he ought to live; and that no general rule can be laid down, which will be equally suitable to all mankind." It should be obvious, after but a moment's reflection, that if this statement were true, our knowledge of how best to live could come only after an extensive personal experience, hence at the end of a life, largely, perhaps, misspent. It would come too late to do us any good. If there are no principles of physiology and biology that are applicable to all of us, if there are no *hy-gienic* practices that are equally good for every man, if every man is a law unto himself, so that what is one man's boon is another man's bane, then there can be no science of health, no possibility of ever learning how to live, except at the end of a long and costly period of personal experience. We would, then, be most likely to kill ourselves in trying to learn to live.

The theory as expressed in Graham's day, and as held today, is that, because there are differences in *constitution, temperament, predisposition,* etc., a way of life that is good for one man may prove harmful to another. If this contention is true, then are we indeed living in a reign of chaos rather than one of law and order. Graham quotes the contention of some of the people of his time that, "Some, with great regularity of habits, and temperance in diet, enjoy good health and live to great age, while others pursuing the same course, are always sickly, and die young; and, on the other hand, some, with great irregularity and intemperance, enjoy health and live to become very old. Therefore what is best for one man, may not be for another; consequently it would be impossible to prescribe any mode of living, which would be suitable to all constitutions and circumstances."

A very hasty and superficial view of the subject lends to this view the appearance of plausibility, but superficial views are never trustworthy. An honest, candid and full investigation of the subject of life and living in their relations to health, disease and length of life, will lead to a different view and to very different conclusions. For, if we go beneath the surface we shall discover the reign of law and order in the realm of life.

Graham's reply to this popular belief was that the person of good constitution who lived a temperate and sober life would enjoy good health to a ripe old age; whereas the person of feeble constitution would be less healthy and live less long. On the other hand the person with strong constitution whose life contains much that is conducive to good health, will live to advanced age despite irregularities, while the person of poor constitution who lives an irregular and decidedly unwholesome life will die young. There would seem to be no contradiction in this. As nobody's life is all bad, there being different degrees of *good* and *bad* in the mixture, length of life must be measured by the rapidity with which the life breaks down and destroys the original constitutional endowment, be it sound and vigorous or unsound and feeble. But the feeble constitution and the vigorous constitution are governed by the same laws of life. There is no logical reason why two constitutions of the same excellence shall endure to the same length of life and in the same condition of health, if one of them is treated kindly and the other abused unmercifully.

The example of Cornaro is an interesting lesson for us in that it reveals to us in dramatic fashion the fact that, even after a life of dissipation and abuse has greatly broken an originally good constitution and brought its possessor within sight of the grim reaper, a complete reversal of the ways of life, a revolution in habits, may result in such restoration of health as to prolong life in usefulness, happiness and strength for many more years. Whatever may be our view of life, we certainly cannot contend that had Cornaro continued on in his dissolute way of life, he would have regained his health and lived to the age he did. There is no reason to doubt that the prognosis of his physicians would have proved reasonably accurate had he not revolutionized his way of life. Drink, gluttony, a dissolute life — these never restored health nor repaired an already greatly impaired constitution. Even small improvements in the way of life are often enough to account for improved health. Certainly no increase in the drinking, gluttony, dissolution, etc., can produce other than harm.

Unfortunately, when we offer such examples as that of Cornaro (there is the other famous one of Jenkins), people generally conclude that, where the examples are so rare, they must be accounted for upon the basis of some accidental or adventitious influence, such as parentage or fortunate circumstances. They are not yet ready to understand that what we know to be true of one man is an example in the strictest sense of the controlling power of the mode of life (Cornaro's life gives us an example of the results of two ways of life) in determining the quality and length of each individual life. Their incredulity, when such matters are presented to them, is the outgrowth of their ignorance and of the fact that they have not yet learned an abiding faith in great principles.

But the examples are not so rare as may at first thought be assumed. That Cornaro's example has received more publicity than that of any other man is, perhaps, true. Thousands of such example, however, have existed and do exist, that have never been publicized. The fact, then, that the *average* man is possessed of nothing more than the vaguest and generally incorrect views of the *modus operandi* of causes operating in the lives of people, is not ground for accepting his erroneous conclusions about the relative merits of opposites mode of living — the two modes being variously blended in the lives of most people. Viewed as cause and effect, opposite modes of life cannot produce identical results and only first-class habits of living can logically be expected to produce superior results.

Certainly the thousands of examples of the saving potency of a hygienic life should be sufficient to awaken men and women to an understanding of the importance of a correct mode of living and arouse in them a desire to be freed, as much as possible, from the uncertainties of a mode of life that is based on no correct principle, the practices of which are irregular and haphazard, and is so plainly unsuccessful. If the presentation of a new edition of Cornaro's famous *treatise* will help in achieving this desirable awakening, it will have served a very useful purpose. Although at the time he wrote, Cornaro could have had nothing but the crudest notions of physiology and pathology, his example of the influences of the two modes of living is not crude and it should be emphasized that thousands who have read his *discourses* have adopted his mode of temperance and abstinence and have been greatly improved in health.

THE FIRST DISCOURSE

ON A TEMPERATE AND HEALTHFUL LIFE

IT is universally agreed, that custom, in time, becomes a second nature, forcing men to use that, whether good or bad, to which they have been habituated; in fact, we see habit, in many instances, gain the ascendancy over reason. This is so undeniably true, that virtuous men, by keeping company with wicked, often fall into the same vicious course of life. Seeing and considering all this, I have decided to write on the vice of intemperance in eating and drinking.

Now, though all are agreed that intemperance is the parent of gluttony, and sober living the offspring of absteminousness; yet, owing to the power of custom, the former is considered a virtue, and the latter as mean and avaricious; and so many men are blinded and besotted to such a degree, that they come to the age of forty or fifty, burdened with strange and painful infirmities, which render them decrepit and useless; whereas, had they lived temperately and soberly, they would in all probability have been sound and hearty, to the age of eighty and upward. To remedy

23

this state of things, it is requisite that men should
live up to the simplicity dictated by nature, which
teaches us to be content with little, and accustom
ourselves to eat no more than is absolutely necessary to support life, remembering that all excess
causes disease and leads to death. How many friends
of mine, men of the finest understanding and most
amiable disposition, have I seen carried off in the
flower of their manhood by reason of excess and over-
feeding, who, had they been temperate, would now be
living, and ornaments to society, and whose company
I should enjoy with as much pleasure as I am now
deprived of it with concern.

In order, therefore, to put a stop to so great an
evil, I have resolved, in this short discourse, to demon-
strate that intemperance is an abuse which may be
removed, and that the good old sober living may be
substituted in its stead; and this I undertake the
more readily, as many young men of the best understanding have urged upon me its necessity because
of many of their parents having died in middle life,
while I remain so sound and hearty at the age of
eighty-one. These young men express a desire to
reach the same term, nature not forbidding us to wish
for longevity; and old age, being, in fact, that time
of life in which prudence can be best exercised, and
the fruits of all the other virtues enjoyed with the

least opposition, the senses then being so subdued, that man gives himself up entirely to reason. They besought me to let them know the method pursued by me to attain it; and then, finding them intent on so laudable a pursuit, I resolved to treat of that method, in order to be of service, not only to them, but to all those who may be willing to peruse this discourse.

I shall therefore give my reasons for renouncing intemperance and betaking myself to a sober course of life, and declare freely the method pursued by me for that purpose, and then show the good effect upon me; from whence it will be seen how easy it is to remove the abuse of free living. I shall conclude, by showing the many conveniences and blessings of temperate life.

I say, then, that the heavy train of infirmities which had made great inroads on my constitution, were my motives for renouncing intemperance, in the matter of too freely eating and drinking, to which I had been addicted, so that, in consequence of it, my stomach became disordered, and I suffered much pain from colic and gout, attended by that which was still worse, an almost continual slow fever, a stomach generally out of order, and a perpetual thirst. From these disorders, the best delivery I had to hope was death.

Finding myself, therefore, between my thirty-fifth and fortieth year in such unhappy circumstances, and having tried everything that could be thought of to relieve me, but to no purpose, the physicians gave me to understand that there was one method left to get the better of my complaints, provided I would resolve to use it, and patiently persevere. This was to live a strictly sober and regular life, which would be of the greatest efficacy; and that of this I might convince myself, since, by my disorders I was become infirm, though not reduced so low but that a regular life might still recover me. They further added, that, if I did not at once adopt this method of strict living, I should in a few months receive no benefit from it, and that in a few more I must resign myself to death.

These arguments made such an impression on me, that, mortified as I was, besides, by the thought of dying in the prime of life, though at the same time perpetually tormented by various diseases, I immediately resolved, in order to avoid at once both disease and death, to betake myself to a regular course of life. Having upon this inquired of them what rules I should follow, they told me that I must only use food, solid or liquid, such as is generally prescribed to sick persons; and both sparingly. These directions, to say the truth, they had before given

Prescription

me, but I had been impatient of such restraint, and had eaten and drank freely of those things I had desired. But, when I had once resolved to live soberly, and according to the dictates of reason, feeling it was my duty as a man so to do, I entered with so much resolution upon this new course of life, that nothing since has been able to divert me from it. The consequence was, that in a few days I began to perceive that such a course agreed well with me; and, by pursuing it, I found myself in less than a year (some people, perhaps, will not believe it) entirely freed from all my complaints.

Having thus recovered my health, I began seriously to consider the power of temperance: if it had efficacy enough to subdue such grievous disorders as mine it must also have power to preserve me in health and strengthen my bad constitution. I therefore applied myself diligently to discover what kinds of food suited me best.

But, first, I resolved to try whether those which pleased my palate were agreeable to my stomach, so that I might judge of the truth of the proverb, which is so universally held, namely:—That, whatever pleases the palate, must agree with the stomach, or, that whatever is palatable must be wholesome and nourishing. The issue was, that I found it to be false, for I soon found that many things which pleased my palate, disagreed with my stomach. Having thus convinced myself that the proverb in question was false, I gave over the use of such meats and wines as did not suit me, and chose those which by experience I found agreed well with me, taking *only as much* as I could easily digest, having strict regard to *quantity* as well as quality; and contrived matters so as never to cloy my stomach with eating or drinking, and always rose from the table with a disposition to eat and drink more. In this I conformed to the proverb, which says, that a man to consult his health must check his appetite. Having in this manner conquered intemperance I betook myself entirely to a temperate and regular life, and this it was which effected in me that alteration already mentioned, that is, in less than a year, it rid me of all those disorders which had taken such hold on me, and which appeared at the time incurable. It had likewise this other good effect, that I no longer experienced those annual fits of sickness, with which I used to be afflicted while I followed my ordinary free manner of eating and drinking. I also became exceedingly healthy, as I have continued from that time to this day; and for no other reason than that I *never* transgressed against regularity and strict moderation.

In consequence, therefore, of my taking such methods, I have always enjoyed, and, God be praised, still

enjoy, the best of health.   It is true, that, besides
the two most important rules relative to eating and
drinking, which I have ever been very scrupulous to
observe (that is, not to take of either, more than my
stomach could easily digest, and to use only those
things which agree with me), I have carefully avoided,
as far as possible, all extreme heat, cold, extraordi-
nary fatigue, interruption of my usual hours of rest,
or staying long in bad air.   I likewise did all that lay
in my power, to avoid those evils, which we do not
find it so easy to remove: melancholy, hatred, and
other violent passions, which appear to have the
greatest influence on our bodies.   I have not, however, been able to guard so well against these disorders, as not to suffer myself now and then to be
hurried away by them.   But I have discovered this
fact, that these passions, have, in the main, no great
influence over bodies governed by the two foregoing
rules of eating and drinking.   Galen, who was an
eminent physician, has said, that, so long as he followed these two rules, he suffered but little from such
disorders, so little, that they never gave him above
a day's uneasiness.   That what he says is true, I am
a living witness, and so are many others who know
me, and have seen me, how often I have been exposed
to heats and colds, and disagreeable changes of
weather, without taking harm, and have likewise seen

me (owing to various misfortunes which have more
than once befallen me) greatly disturbed in mind;
these things, however, did me but little harm, whereas,
other members of my family, who followed not my
way of living, were greatly disturbed; such in a
word, was their grief and dejection at seeing me in-
volved in expensive law suits, commenced against me
by great and powerful men, that, fearing I should be
ruined, they were seized with great melancholy humor, with which intemperate bodies always abound,
and such influence had it over their bodies, that they
were carried off before their time; whereas, I suffered nothing on the occasion, as I had in me no
superfluous humors of that kind; nay, in order to
keep up my spirits, I brought myself to think that
God had permitted these suits against me, in order to
make me more sensible of my strength of body and
mind; and that I should get the better of them with
honor and advantage, as it, in fact, came to pass;
for, at last, I obtained a decree exceedingly favorable
to my fortune and character.

But I may go a step farther, and show how favorable to recovery is a temperate life, in case of
accident. At the age of seventy years, I happened,
as is often the case, to be in a coach, which, going
at a smart rate, was upset, and in that condition
drawn a considerable way before the horses could

be stopped. I received so many shocks and bruises, that I was taken out with my head and body terribly battered, and a dislocated leg and arm. When the physicians saw me in so bad a plight, they concluded that in three days I should die, but thought they would try what bleeding and purging would do, in order to prevent inflammation and fever. But I, on the contrary, knowing that, by reason of the sober life I had lived for so many years, my blood was in good and pure condition, refused to be either purged or bled. I just caused my arm and leg to be set, and suffered myself to be rubbed with some oils, which they said were proper on the occasion. Thus, without using any other kind of remedy, I recovered, as I thought I should, without feeling the least alteration in myself, or any bad effects from the accident; a thing which appeared no less than miraculous in the eyes of the physicians. Hence, we may infer, that he who leads a sober and regular life, and commits no excess in his diet, can suffer but little from mental disorders or external accidents. On the contrary, I conclude, especially from the late trial I have had, that excesses in eating and drinking are often fatal. Four years ago, I consented to increase the quantity of my food by two ounces, my friends and relations having, for some time past, urged upon me the necessity of such increase, that the quantity I

took was too little for one so advanced in years;
against this, I urged that nature was content with
little, and that with this small quantity I had pre-
served myself for many years in health and activity,
that I believed as a man advanced in years, his stomach grew weaker, and therefore the tendency should
be to lessen the amount of food rather than to increase. I further reminded them of the two proverbs,
which say: he who has a mind to eat a great deal,
must eat but little; eating little makes life long, and,
living long, he must eat much; and the other proverb
was: that, what we *leave* after making a hearty meal,
does us more good than what we have eaten. But my
arguments and proverbs were not able to prevent
them teasing me upon the subject; therefore, not to
appear obstinate, or affecting to know more than the
physicians themselves, but above all, to please my
family, I consented to the increase before mentioned;
so that, whereas previous, what with bread, meat, the
yolk of an egg, and soup, I ate as much as twelve
ounces, neither more nor less, I now increased it to
fourteen; and whereas before I drank but fourteen
ounces of wine, I now increased it to sixteen. This
increase, had, in eight days' time, such an effect upon
me, that, from being cheerful and brisk, I began to
be peevish and melancholy, so that nothing could
please me. On the twelfth day, I was attacked with a

violent pain in my side, which lasted twenty-two
hours and was followed by a fever, which continued
thirty-five days without any respite, insomuch that
all looked upon me as a dead man; but, God be
praised, I recovered, and I am positive that it was
the great regularity I had observed for so many
years, and that only, which rescued me from the jaws
of death.

Orderly living is, doubtless, a most certain cause
and foundation of health and long life; nay, I say it
is the only true medicine, and whoever weighs the matter well, will come to this conclusion. Hence it is,
that when the physician comes to visit a patient, the
first thing he prescribes is regular living, and certainly to avoid excess. Now, if the patient after recovery should continue so to live, he could not be
sick again, and if a very small quantity of food is
sufficient to restore his health, then but a slight addi-
tion is necessary for the continuance of the same;
and so, for the future, he would want neither physician nor physic. Nay, by attending to what I have
said, he would become his own physician, and indeed, the best he could have, since, in fact, no man
should be a perfect physician to any but himself.
The reason is, that any man, by repeated trials, may
acquire a perfect knowledge of his own constitution,
the kinds of food and drink which agree with him

best. These repeated trials are necessary, as there is a great variety in the nature and stomachs of persons. I found that old wine did not suit me, but that the new wines did; and, after long practice, I discovered that many things, which might not be injurious to others, were not good for me. Now, where is the physician who could have informed me which to take, and which to avoid, since I by long observation, could scarce discover these things.

It follows, therefore, that it is impossible to be a perfect physician to another. A man cannot have a better guide than himself, nor any physic better than a regular life. I do not, however, mean that for the knowledge and cure of such disorders as befall those who live an irregular life there is no occasion for a physician and that his assistance ought to be slighted; such persons should at once call in medical aid, in case of sickness. But, for the bare purpose of keeping ourselves in good health, I am of opinion, that we should consider this regular life as our physician, since it preserves men, even those of a weak constitution, in health; makes them live sound and hearty, to the age of one hundred and upward, and prevents their dying of sickness, or through the corruption of their humors, but merely by the natural decay, which at the last must come to all. These things, however, are discovered but by few, for men, for the most part, are sensual and intemperate, and love to satisfy their appetites, and to commit every excess; and, by way of apology, say that they prefer a short and self-indulgent life, to a long and self-denying one, not knowing that those men are most truly happy who keep their appetites in subjection. Thus have I found it, and I prefer to live temperately, so that I may live long and be useful. Had I not been temperate, I should never have written these tracts, which I have the pleasure of thinking will be serviceable to others. Sensual men affirm that no man can live a regular life. To this I answer, that Galen, who was a great physician, led such a life, and chose it as the best physic. The same did Plato, Cicero, Isocrates, and many other great men of former times, whom not to tire the reader I forbear naming; and, in our days, Pope Paul Farnese and Cardinal Bembo; and it was for that reason they lived so long. Therefore, since many have led this life, and many are actually leading it, surely all might conform to it, and the more so, as no great difficulty attends it. Cicero affirms that nothing is needed, but to be in good earnest. Plato, you say, though he himself lived thus regularly, affirms that, in republics, men often cannot do so, being obliged to expose themselves to various hardships and changes, which are incompatible with a regular life. I answer, that men

who have to undergo these things, would be the better
able to bear such hardships by being strictly temperate in matters of eating and drinking.

Here it may be objected, that he who leads this
strict and regular life, having constantly when well
made use only of simple food fit for the sick, and in
small quantities, has when himself in sickness, no re-
course left in matters of diet. To which I reply,
that, whoever leads a regular life, cannot be sick or
at least but seldom. By a regular life I mean, that
a man shall ascertain for himself, how small a quantity of food and drink is sufficient to supply the daily
wants of his nature and then having done this, and
found out the kinds of food and drink best suited for
his constitution, he shall, having formed his plans,
strictly adhere to his resolutions and principles, not
being careful at one time, and self-indulgent at others,
for by so doing, he would gain but little benefit; but
taking care always to avoid excess, which any man
can certainly do at all times, and under all circumstances, if he is determined. I say then, that he who
thus lives cannot be sick, or but seldom, and for a
short time, because, by regular living, he destroys
every seed of sickness, and thus, by removing the
cause, prevents the effect; so that he who pursues a
regular and strictly moderate life, need not fear
illness, for his blood having become pure, and free

Humors = Body Fluid i.e., Blood or Bile

from all bad humors, it is not possible that he can
fall sick.

Since, therefore, it appears that a regular life is
so profitable and virtuous, it ought to be universally
followed; and more so, as it does not clash with du-
ties of any kind, but is easy to all. Neither is it necessary that all should eat as little as I do—twelve
ounces—or not to eat of many things from which I,
because of the natural weakness of my stomach, ab-
stain. Those with whom all kinds of food agree,
may eat of such, only they are forbidden to eat a
greater quantity, even of that which agrees with them
best, than their stomachs can with ease digest. The
same is to be understood of drink. The only rule
for such to observe in eating and drinking, is the
quantity rather than the quality; but for those who,
like myself, are weak of constitution, these must not
only be careful as to quantity, but also to quality,
partaking only of such things as are simple, and easy
to digest.

Let no one tell me that there are numbers, who,
though they live most irregularly, attain in health
and spirits to a great age. This argument is
grounded on uncertainty and hazard, and such cases
are rare. Men should not, therefore, because of these
exceptional cases, be persuaded to irregularity or
indulgence. Whoever, trusting to the strength of

his constitution, slights these observations, may expect to suffer by so doing, and to live in constant danger of disease and death. I therefore affirm, that a man, even of a bad constitution, who leads a strictly regular and sober life, is surer of a long one, than he of the best constitution who lives carelessly and irregularly. If men have a mind to live long and healthy, and die without sickness of body or mind, but by mere dissolution, they must submit to a regular and abstemious life, for such a life keeps the blood clean and pure. It suffers no vapors to ascend from the stomach to the head; hence, the brain of him who thus lives enjoys constant serenity; he can soar above the low and groveling concerns of this life to the exalted and beautiful contemplation of heavenly things to his exceeding comfort and satisfaction. He then truly discerns the brutality of those excesses into which men fall, and which bring them misery here and hereafter; while he may with comfort look forward to a long life, conscious that, through the mercy of God, he has relinquished the paths of vice and intemperance, never again to enter them; and, through the merits of our Saviour Jesus Christ, to die in His favor. He therefore does not suffer himself to be cast down with the thoughts of death, knowing that it will not attack him violently, or by surprise, or with sharp pains and feverish sensations, but will come upon him with ease and gentleness; like a lamp, the oil of which is exhausted, he will pass gently, and without any sickness, from this terrestrial and mortal, to a celestial and eternal life.

Some sensual unthinking persons affirm, that a long life is no great blessing, and that the state of a man, who has passed his seventy-fifth year, cannot really be called life; but this is wrong, as I shall fully prove; and it is my sincere wish, that all men would endeavor to attain my age, that they might enjoy that period of life, which of all others is most desirable.

I will therefore give an account of my recreations, and the relish which I find at this stage of life. There are many who can give testimony as to the happiness of my life. In the first place, they see with astonishment the good state of my health and spirits; how I mount my horse without assistance, how I not only ascend a flight of stairs, but can climb a hill with greatest ease. Then, how gay and good-humored I am; my mind ever undisturbed, in fact, joy and peace having fixed their abode in my breast. Moreover, they know in what manner I spend my time, so as never to find life weary: I pass my hours in great delight and pleasure, in converse with men of good sense and intellectual culture; then, when I cannot enjoy their company, I betake myself to the reading

of some good book. When I have read as much as I
like, I write; endeavoring in this, as in other things
to be of service to others; and these things I do with
the greatest ease to myself, living in a pleasant house
in the most beautiful quarter of this noble city of
Padua. Besides this house, I have my gardens, supplied with pleasant streams in which I always find
something to do which amuses me. Nor are my recreations rendered less agreeable by the failing of any
of my senses, for they are all, thank God, perfect,
particularly my palate, which now relishes better the
simple fare I have, than it formerly did the most
delicate dishes, when I led an irregular life. Nor
does the change of beds give me any uneasiness: I
can sleep everywhere soundly and quietly, and my
dreams are pleasant and delightful. It is likewise
with the greatest pleasure I behold the success of an
undertaking so important to this state; I mean that
of draining and improving so many uncultivated
pieces of ground, an undertaking begun within my
memory, but which I thought I should never see com-
pleted; nevertheless I have, and was even in person
assisting in the work for two months together, in
those marshy places during the heats in summer,
without ever finding myself worse for the fatigues or
inconveniences I suffered; of so much efficacy is that
orderly life, which I everywhere constantly lead.

Such are some of the recreations and diversions of
my old age, which is so much the more to be valued
than the old age, or even the youth of other men; as,
being freed by God's grace from the perturbations
of the mind and the infirmities of the body, I no
longer experience any of those contrary emotions
which rack such a number of young men and as many
old ones, who, by reason of their careless living
and intemperate habits, are destitute of health and
strength, and consequently of all true enjoyment.

And if it be lawful to compare little matters to
affairs of importance, I will further venture to say,
that such are the effects of this sober life, that, at my
present age of eighty-three, I have been able to write
an entertaining comedy, abounding with innocent
mirth and pleasant jests.

I have yet another comfort which I will mention;
that of seeing a kind of immortality in a succession
of descendants; for, as often as I return home, I
find before me, not one or two, but eleven grandchildren, the oldest of them eighteen, all the offspring of
one father and mother, and all blessed with good
health.   Some of the youngest I play with; those
older, I make companions of; and, as nature has be-
stowed good voices upon them, I amuse myself by
hearing them sing, and play on different instruments.
Nay, I sing myself, as I have a better voice now,

clearer and louder, than at any period of my life. Such are the recreations of my old age.

Whence it appears, that the life I lead is not gloomy, but cheerful, and I would not exchange my manner of living and my gray hairs, with that of even a young man, having the best constitution, who gave way to his appetites; knowing, as I do, that such are daily subject to a thousand kinds of ailments and death. I remember my own conduct in early life, and I know how foolhardy are young men; how apt they are to presume on their strength in all their actions, and by reason of their little experience, are oversanguine in their expectations. Hence, they often expose themselves rashly to every kind of danger, and, banishing reason, bow their necks to the yoke of concupiscence, and endeavor to gratify all their appetites, not minding, fools as they are, that they thereby hasten the approach of what they would most willingly avoid, sickness and death.

And these are two great evils to all men who live a free life; the one is troublesome and painful, the other, dreadful and insupportable, especially when they reflect on the errors to which this mortal life is subject, and on the vengeance which the justice of God is wont to take on sinners. Whereas, I, in my old age, praise to the Almighty, am exempt from these torments; from the first, because I cannot fall

sick, having removed all the cause of illness by my
regularity and moderation; from the other, that of
death, because from so many years' experience, I
have learned to obey reason; whereas, I not only think
it a great folly to fear that which cannot be avoided,
but likewise firmly expect some consolation, from the
grace of Jesus Christ, when I arrive at that period.

But though I know I must, like others, reach that
term, it is yet at so great a distance that I cannot
discern it, because *I know I shall not die except by
mere dissolution*, having already, by my regular
course of life, shut up all other avenues of death,
and thus prevented the humors of my body making
any other war upon me, than that which I must expect from the elements employed in the composition
of this mortal frame.   I am not so simple as not to
know that, as I was born, so I must die; but the
natural death that I speak of does not overtake one,
until after a long course of years; and even then, I
do not expect the pain and agony which most men
suffer when they die.   But I, by God's blessing,
reckon that I have still a long time to live in health
and spirits, and enjoy this beautiful world, which is,
indeed, beautiful to those who know how to make it
so, but its beauty can only be realized by those who,
by reason of temperance and virtue, enjoy sound
health of body and mind.

Now, if this sober and moderate manner of living brings so much happiness; if the blessings that attend it are so stable and permanent, then I beseech every man of sound judgment to embrace this valuable treasure, that of a long and healthful life, a treasure which exceeds all other worldly blessings, and, therefore, should be sought after; for what is wealth and abundance to a man who is possessed with a feeble and sickly body? This is that divine sobriety, agreeable to God, the friend of nature, the daughter of reason, the sister of all the virtues, the companion of temperate living, modest, courteous, content with little, regular, and perfectly mistress of all her operations. From her, as from their proper root, spring life, health, cheerfulness, industry, learning and all those actions and employments worthy of noble and generous minds. The laws of God are all in her favor. Repletion, excess, intemperance, superfluous humors, diseases, fevers, pains, and the dangers of death, vanish in her presence, as mists before the sun. Her comeliness ravishes every well-disposed mind. Her influence is so sure, as to promise to all a long and agreeable life. And, lastly, she promises to be a mild and pleasant guardian of life, teaching how to ward off the attacks of death. Strict sobriety, in eating and drinking, renders the senses and understanding clear, the memory tenacious, the body lively and strong, the movements regular and easy; and the soul, feeling so little of her earthly burden, experiences much of her natural liberty. The man thus enjoys a pleasing and agreeable harmony, there being nothing in his system to disturb; for his blood is pure, and runs freely through his veins, and the heat of his body is mild and temperate.

SHOWING THE SUREST METHOD OF COR-
RECTING AN INFIRM CONSTITUTION

My treatise on a sober life has begun to answer
my desire, in being of service to many persons born
of a weak constitution, or who, by reason of free living, have become infirm, who, when they commit the
least excess, find themselves greatly indisposed. I
should also be glad to be of service to those, who,
born with a good constitution, yet, by reason of a
disorderly life, find themselves at the age of fifty or
sixty attacked with various pains and diseases, such
as gout, sciatica, liver and stomach complaints, to
which they would not be subject, were they to live a
strictly temperate life, and by so doing would moreover greatly increase the term of their existence, and
live with much greater comfort; they would find
themselves less irritable, and less disposed to be upset
by inconvenience and annoyance. I was myself of a
most irritable disposition, insomuch that at times
there was no living with me. Now, for a very long
time it has been otherwise, and I can see that a person swayed by his passions is little or no better than
a madman at such times.

46

The man, also, who is of a *bad* constitution, may, by dint of reason, and a regular and sober life, live to a great age and in good health, as I have done, who had naturally one of the worst, so that it appeared impossible I should live above forty years, whereas, I now find myself sound and hearty at the age of eighty-six; forty-six years beyond the time I had expected; and during this long respite all my senses have continued perfect; and even my teeth, my voice, my memory, and my heart.. But what is still more, my brain is clearer now than it ever was. Nor do any of my powers abate as I advance in life; and this because, as I grow older, I lessen the quantity of my solid food. This retrenchment is necessary, since it is impossible for man to live for ever; and, as he draws near his end, he is brought so low as to be able to take but little nourishment, and at such times, the yolk of an egg, and a few spoonfuls of milk with bread, is quite sufficient during the twenty-four hours; a greater quantity would most likely cause pain, and shorten life. In my own case, I expect to die without any pain or sickness, and this is a blessing of great importance; yet may be expected by those who shall lead a sober life, whether they be rich or poor. And, since a long and healthy life ought to be greatly coveted by every man, then I conclude that all men are in duty bound to exert themselves to that effect; nevertheless such a blessing cannot be obtained without strict temperance and sobriety. But some allege that many, without leading such a life, have lived to a hundred, and that in good health, though they ate a great deal, and used indiscriminately every kind of viands and wine, and therefore they flatter themselves that they shall be equally fortunate. But in this they are guilty of two mistakes: the first is, that it is not one in fifty thousand that ever attains that happiness; the other mistake is, that such, in the end, most certainly contract some illness, which carries them off: nor can they be sure of ending their days otherwise; so that the safest way to attain a long and healthful life, is to embrace sobriety, and to diet oneself strictly as to quantity. And this is no very difficult affair. History informs us of many who lived in the greatest temperance; and this present age furnishes us with many such, reckoning myself one of the number: we are all human beings, endowed with reason, and consequently we ought to be master of all our actions.

This sobriety is reduced to two things, quality and quantity. The first consists in avoiding food or drinks, which are found to *disagree* with the stomach. The second, to avoid taking more than the stomach can easily *digest*; and every man at the age of forty ought to be a perfect judge in these matters; and

whoever observes these two rules, may be said to live
a regular and sober life. And the virtue and efficacy
of this life is such, that the humors in a man's blood
become harmonious and perfect, and are no longer
liable to be disturbed or corrupted by any disorders,
such as suffering from excessive heat or cold, too
much fatigue, or want of rest, and the like. A man
who lives as I have described, may pass through all
these changes without harm. Wherefore, since the
humors of persons who observe these two rules relative to eating and drinking, cannot possibly be corrupted and engender acute diseases (the cause of untimely death), every man is bound to comply with
them, for whoever acts otherwise, living a disorderly
life, instead of a regular one, is constantly exposed
to disease and death.

It is, indeed, true that even those who observe the
two rules relating to diet, the observance of which
constitutes a regular life, may, by committing any
one of the other irregularities, such as excessive heat,
cold, fatigue, etc., find himself slightly indisposed for
a day or two, but he need fear nothing worse.

But as there are some persons who, though well
stricken in years, are, nevertheless, very free in their
living, and allege that neither the quantity nor the
quality of their diet makes any impression upon
them, and therefore eat a great deal of everything

without distinction, and indulge themselves equally in point of drinking; such men are ignorant of the requirements of their nature, or they are gluttonous; and I do affirm, that such do not enjoy good health, but as a rule are infirm, irritable, and full of maladies. There are others, who say that it is necessary that they should eat and drink freely to keep up their natural heat, which is constantly diminishing, as they advance in years; and that it is therefore their duty to eat heartily of such things as please their palate, and that strict moderation, in their case, would tend to shorten life. Now, this is the reason, or excuse, of thousands. But to all this, I answer, that all such are deceiving themselves, and I speak from experience, as well as observation. The fact is, large quantities of food cannot be digested by old stomachs; as man gets weaker as he grows older, and the waste in his system is slower, the natural heat certainly is less. Nor will all the food in the world increase it, except to bring on fever and distressing disorders; therefore, let none be afraid of shortening their days by eating too little. I am strong and hearty, and full of good spirits, neither have I ache or pain, and yet I am very old, and subsist upon very little; and, in this respect, that which would suit one man, is good for another. When men are taken ill they discontinue, or nearly so, their food. Now, if by reducing themselves to a small quantity, they recover from the jaws of death, how can they doubt, but that, with a slight increase of diet consistent with reason, they will be able to support nature, when in health. Let a fair, honest trial of some few weeks be given, and the result would, in all cases, be most pleasing.

Others say, that it is better for a man to suffer three or four times every year, from gout, sciatica, or whatever disorder to which he may be subject, than be tormented the whole year by not indulging his appetite, and eating and drinking just as he pleases, since he can always by a few days of self-denial recover from all such attacks. To this I answer, that, our natural heat growing less and less as we advance in years, no abstinence for a *short time* can have virtue sufficient to conquer the malady to which the man is subject, and which is generally brought on by repletion, so that he must die at last of one of these periodical disorders; for they abridge life in the same proportion as temperance and health prolong it.

Others pretend that it is better to live a short and self-indulgent life, than a long and self-denying one; but surely, longevity ought to be valued, and is, by men of good understanding; and those who do not truly prize this great gift of God, are surely a disgrace to mankind, and their death is a service to the public rather than not. And again, there are some, who, though they are conscious that they become weaker as they advance in years, yet cannot be brought to retrench the quantity of their food, but rather increase it, and, because they find themselves unable to digest the great quantity of food, with which they load their stomachs twice or thrice a day, they resolve to eat but once, heartily, in the twenty-four hours. But this course is useless; for the stomach is still overburdened, and the food is not digested, but turns into bad humors, by which the blood becomes poisoned, and thus a man kills himself long before his time. I never met with an aged person who enjoyed health, and lived that manner of life. Now, all these men whose manner of life I have named, would live long and happily, if, as they advanced in years, they lessened the *quantity* of their food, and ate oftener, and but little at a time, for old stomachs cannot digest large quantities, men at this age becoming children again, who eat little and often during the twenty-four hours.

O thrice holy sobriety, so useful to man, by reason of the service thou dost render him! Thou prolongest his days, by which means he greatly improves his understanding and, by such knowledge, he can avoid the bitter fruits of sensuality, which is an enemy to man's reason. Thou, moreover, freest him from the dreadful thoughts of death. How greatly ought we to be indebted to thee, since by thee we enjoy this beautiful world, which is really beautiful to all whose sensibilities have not been deadened by repletion, and whose minds have not been blighted by sensuality! I really never knew till I grew old, that the world was so beautiful; for, in my younger years I was debauched by irregularities, and therefore could not perceive and enjoy, as I do now, its beauties. O truly happy life, which, over and above all these favors conferred on me, hast so improved and perfected my body, that now I have a better relish for plain bread, than formerly I had for the most exquisite dainties! in fact I find such sweetness in it, because of the good appetite I always have, that I should be afraid of sinning against temperance, were I not convinced of the absolute necessity for it, and knowing that pure bread is, above all things, man's best food, and while he leads a sober life, he may be sure of never wanting that natural sauce,—a good appetite—and moreover, I find that, whereas I used to eat twice a day, now that I am much older, it is better for me to eat four times, and still to lessen the quantity as the years increase. And this is what I do, guided by my experience; therefore, my spirits being never oppressed by too much food, are always brisk; especially after eating, so that I enjoy much

Repletion = Plentifully Supplied, Abounding, Filled to Satiation, Gorged

the singing of a song, before I sit down to my writing.

Nor do I ever find myself the worse for writing directly after meals; my understanding is never clearer; and I am never drowsy; the food I take being too small a quantity to send up any fumes to the brain. O, how advantageous it is to an old man to eat but little; therefore I take but just enough to keep body and soul together, and the things I eat are as follows: bread, panado, eggs (the yolk), and soups. Of flesh meat, I eat kid and mutton. I eat poultry of every kind; also of sea and river fish. Some men are too poor to allow themselves food of this kind, but they may do well on bread (made from wheat meal, which contains far more nutriment than bread made from fine flour), panado, eggs, milk, and vegetables. But though a man should eat nothing but these, he may not eat more than his stomach can with ease digest, never forgetting that it is the over-quantity which injures, even more than the eating of unsuitable food. And again I say, that whoever does not transgress, in point of either quantity or quality, cannot die, but by mere dissolution, except in cases where there is some inherited disease to combat; but such cases are comparatively rare, and even here a strict and sober diet will be of the greatest service.

O, what a difference between a regular and temperate life, and an irregular and intemperate life!

One gives health and longevity, the other produces
disease and untimely death. How many of my dear-
est relations and friends have I lost by their free
living, whereas, had they listened to me, they might
have been full of life and health. I am thus more
than ever determined to use my utmost endeavors to
make known the benefit of my kind of life. Here I
am, an old man, yet full of life and joy, happier than
at any previous period of my life, surrounded by
many comforts; not the least to mention are my
eleven grand-children, all of fine understanding and
amiable disposition, beautiful in their persons, and
well disposed to learning; and these, I hope so to
teach, that they shall take pattern after me, and
follow my kind of life.

Now, I am often at a loss to understand why men
of fine parts and understanding, who have attained
middle age, do not, when they find themselves attacked
by disorders and sickness, betake themselves to a
regular life, and that constantly. Is it because they
are in ignorance as to the importance of this subject? Surely, it cannot be that they are enslaved
by their appetites to such an extent that they find
themselves unable to adopt a strict and regular diet?
As to young men, I am in no way surprised at their
refusal to live such a life, for their passions are
strong and usually their guide. Neither have they

much experience; but, when a man has arrived at
the age of forty or fifty, surely he should in all
things be governed by reason. And this would teach
men that gratifying the appetite and palate, is not,
as many affirm, natural and right, but is the cause
of disease and premature death. Were this pleasure
of the palate lasting, it would be some excuse; but it
is momentary, compared with the duration of the disease which its excess engenders. But it is a great
comfort to a man of sober life to reflect, that what he
eats will keep him in good health, and be productive
of no disease or infirmity.

THE METHOD OF ENJOYING COMPLETE HAPPINESS IN OLD AGE

MY LORD,

In writing to your Lordship, it is true I shall speak of few things, but such as I have already mentioned in my essays, but I am sure your Lordship will not tire of the repetition.

Now, my Lord, to begin, I must tell you, that being now at the age of ninety-one, I am more sound and hearty than ever, much to the amazement of those who know me. I, who can account for it, am bound to show that a man can enjoy a terrestrial paradise after eighty; but it is not to be obtained, except by strict temperance in food and drink, virtues acceptable to God and friends to reason. I must, however, go on to tell you, that, during the past few days I have been visited by many of the learned doctors of this university, as well as physicians and philosophers who were well acquainted with my age, life, and manners, also, that I was stout, hearty, and lively, my senses perfect, also my voice and teeth, likewise my memory and judgment. They knew, besides, that I constantly employed eight hours every day in writing treatises, with my own hand, on subjects useful to mankind, and spent many more in walking and singing. O, my Lord, how melodious my voice is grown! Were you to hear me chant my prayers, and that to my lyre, after the example of David, I am certain it would give you great pleasure, my voice is so musical.

Now, these doctors and philosophers told me that it was next to a miracle, that at my age, I should be able to write upon subjects which required both judgment and spirit, and added that I ought not to be looked upon as a person advanced in years, since all my occupations were those of a young man, and that I was altogether unlike aged people of seventy and eighty, who are subject to various ailments and diseases, which render life a weariness; or, if even any by chance escape these things, yet their senses are impaired, sight, or hearing, or memory is defective, and all their faculties much decayed; they are not strong, nor cheerful, as I am. And they moreover said, that they looked upon me as having special grace conferred upon me, and said a great many eloquent and fine things, in endeavoring to prove this, which, however, they could not do; for their arguments were not grounded on good and sufficient reasons, but merely on their opinions. I therefore

endeavored to undeceive and set them right, and
convince them that the happiness I enjoyed was not
confined to me, but might be common to all mankind,
since I was but a mere mortal, and different in no
respect from other men, save in this, that I was born
more weakly than some, and had not what is called
a strong constitution. Man, however, in his youthful
days, is more prone to be led by sensuality than reason; yet, when he arrives at the age of forty, or
earlier, he should remember that he has about reached
the summit of the hill, and must now think of going
down, carrying the weight of years with him; and
that old age is the reverse of youth, as much as order
is the reverse of disorder; hence, it is requisite that
he should alter his mode of life, in regard to the
quality and quantity of his food and drink. For it
is impossible in the nature of things, that the man
who is bent on indulging his appetite, should be
healthy and free from ailments. Hence it was to
avoid this vice and its evil effects, I embraced a
regular and sober life. It is no doubt true, that I
at first found some difficulty in accomplishing this,
but in order to conquer the difficulty I besought the
Almighty to grant the virtue of sobriety in all things,
well knowing that He would graciously hear my
prayer. Then, considering that when a man is about
to undertake a thing of importance, which he knows

he can compass, though not without difficulty, he may
make it much easier to himself by being steady in
his purpose, I pursued this course: I endeavored
gradually to relinquish a disorderly life, and to suit
myself to strict temperate rules; and thus it came
to pass, that a sober and moderate life no longer
became disagreeable, though, on account of the weakness of my constitution, I tied myself down to very
strict rules in regard to the quantity and quality
of what I ate and drank.

Others, who happen to be blessed with a strong
constitution, may eat a greater variety of food, and
in somewhat larger quantity, each man being a guide
to himself, consulting always his judgment and reason, rather than his fancy or appetite, and further
let him always strictly abide by his rules, for he
will receive little benefit if he occasionally indulges
in excess.

Now, on hearing these arguments, and examining
the reasons on which they were founded, the doctors
and philosophers agreed that I had advanced nothing
but what was true. One of the younger of them
said that I appeared to enjoy the special grace of
being able to relinquish, with ease, one kind of life,
and embrace another, a thing which he knew from
theory to be feasible, but in practice to be difficult,
for it had proved as hard to him, as easy to me.

To this I replied, that, being human like himself, I likewise had found it no easy task, but it did not become a man to shrink from a glorious and practical task, on account of its difficulties; the greater the obstacles to overcome, the greater the honor and benefit. Our beneficent Creator is desirous, that, as He originally favored human nature with longevity, we should all enjoy the full advantage of His intentions, knowing that when a man has passed seventy, he may be exempt from the sensual strivings, and govern himself entirely by the dictates of reason. Vice and immorality then leave him, and God is willing that he should live to the full maturity of his years, and has ordained that all who reach their natural term should end their days without sickness, but by mere dissolution, the natural way; the wheels of life quietly stopping, and man peacefully leaving this world, to enter upon immortality, as will be my case; for I am sure to die thus, perhaps while chanting my prayers. Nor do the thoughts of death give me the least concern; nor does any other thought connected with death, namely, the fear of the punishment to which wicked men are liable, because I am bound to believe, that being a Christian, I shall be saved by the virtue of the most sacred blood of Jesus Christ, which He freely shed in order to save those who trust in Him. Thus, how beautiful my life!

how happy my end! To this, the young doctor had nothing to reply, but that he would follow my example.

The great desire I had, my Lord, to converse with you at this distance, has forced me to be prolix, and still obliges me to proceed, though not much farther. There are some sensualists, my Lord, who say that I have thrown away my time and trouble, in writing a treatise upon temperance, and other discourses on the same subject; alleging, that it is impossible to conform to it, so that my treatise must answer as little purpose as that of Plato on Government, who took a great deal of pains to recommend a thing impracticable. Now, this much surprises me, as they may see that I lived a sober life many years before I wrote my treatise, and I should never have composed it, had I not been convinced, that it was such a life as any man might lead; and being a virtuous life, would be of great service to him; so that I felt myself under an obligation to present it in its true light. Again, I have the satisfaction to hear that numbers, on reading my treatise, have embraced such a life. So that the objection concerning Plato on Government is of no force against my case. But a sensualist is an enemy to reason, and a slave to his passions.

AN EXHORTATION TO A SOBER AND REGULAR LIFE, IN ORDER TO ATTAIN OLD AGE

NOT to be wanting in my duty, and not to lose at the same time the satisfaction I feel in being useful to others, I again take up my pen to inform those, who, for want of conversing with me, are strangers to what those with whom I am acquainted. know and see. But as some things may appear to certain persons scarcely credible, though actually true, I shall not fail to relate for the benefit of the public. Wherefore, I say, being arrived at my ninety fifth year, God be praised, and still finding myself sound and hearty, content and cheerful, I never cease to thank the Divine Majesty for so great a blessing, considering the usual condition of old men. These scarcely ever attain the age of seventy, without losing health and spirits, and growing melancholy and peevish. Moreover, when I remember how weak and sickly I was between the ages of thirty and forty, and how from the first, I never had what is called a strong constitution; I say, when I remember these things, I have surely abundant cause for gratitude,

63

and though I know I cannot live many years longer, the thought of death gives me no uneasiness; I, moreover, firmly believe that I shall attain to the age of one hundred years. But, to render this dissertation more methodical, I shall begin by considering man at his birth; and from thence accompany him through every stage of life, to his grave.

I therefore say, that some come into the world with the stamina of life so weak, that they live but a few days, or months, or years, and it is not always easy to show, to what the shortness of life is owing. Others are born sound and lively, but still, with a poor, weakly constitution; and of these, some live to the age of ten, twenty, others to thirty or forty, but seldom live to be old men. Others, again, bring into the world a perfect constitution, and live to an old age; but it is generally, as I have said, an old age of sickness and sorrow, for which usually they have to thank themselves, because they unreasonably presumed on the goodness of their constitution; and cannot, by any means, be brought to alter when grown old, from the mode of life they pursued in their younger days, but live as irregularly when past the meridian of life, as they did in the time of their youth. They do not consider, that the stomach has lost much of its natural heat and vigor, and that, therefore, they should pay great attention to the

quality and quantity of what they eat and drink;
but, rather than decrease, many of them are for
increasing the quantity, saying, that, as health and
vigor grow less, they should endeavor to repair the
loss by a great abundance of food, since it is by sus-
tenance we are to preserve ourselves.

But it is here that the great mistake is made; since,
as the natural force and heat lessen as a man grows
in years, he should diminish the quantity of his food
and drink, as nature at that period is content with
little; and moreover, if increasing the amount of
nourishment was the proper thing, then, surely the
majority of men would live to a great age in the
best of health. But do we see it so? On the contrary, such a case is a rare exception; whilst my
course of life is proved to be right, by reason of
its results. But, though some have every reason
to believe this to be the case, they nevertheless, because of their want of strength of character, and
their love of repletion, still continue their usual manner of living. But were they, in due time, to form
strict temperate habits, they would not grow infirm
in their old age, but would continue as I am, strong
and hearty, and might live to the age of one hundred, or one hundred and twenty. This has been
the case with others of whom we read, men who were
born with a good constitution, and lived sober and

abstemious lives; and had it been my lot to have enjoyed a strong constitution, I should make no doubt of attaining to that age. But as I was born feeble, and with an infirm constitution, I am afraid I shall not outlive an hundred years; and were others, born weakly as myself, to betake them to a life like mine, they would, like me, live to the age of a hundred, as shall be my case.

And this certainty of being able to live to a great age is, in my opinion, a great advantage (of course I do not include accidents, to which all are liable, and which must specially be left to our Maker), and highly to be valued; none being sure of this blessing, except such as adhere to the rules of temperance. This security of life is built on good and truly natural reasons, which can never fail; it being impossible that he who leads a perfectly sober and temperate life, should breed any sickness, or die before his time. Sooner, he cannot through ill-health die, as his sober life has the virtue to remove the cause of sickness, and sickness cannot happen without a cause; which cause being removed, sickness is also removed, and untimely and painful death prevented.

And there is no doubt, that temperance in food and drink, taking only as much as nature really requires, and thus being guided by reason, instead of appetite, has efficacy to remove all cause of disease;

for since health and sickness, life and death, depend
on the good or bad condition of a man's blood, and
the quality of his humors, such a life as I speak of
purifies the blood, and corrects all vicious humors,
rendering all perfect and harmonious. It is true,
and cannot be denied, that man must at last die,
however careful with himself he may have been; but
yet, I maintain, without sickness and great pain;
for in my case I expect to pass away quietly and
peacefully, and my present condition insures this
to me, for, though at this great age, I am hearty
and content, eating with a good appetite, and sleep-
ing soundly. Moreover, all my senses are as good
as ever, and in the highest perfection; my understanding clear and bright, my judgment sound, my
memory tenacious, my spirits good, and my voice
(one of the first things which is apt to fail us) has
grown so strong and sonorous, that I cannot help
chanting aloud my prayers, morning and night, instead of whispering and muttering them to myself
as was formerly my custom.

O, how glorious is this life of mine, replete with
all the felicities which man can enjoy on this side
of the grave! It is entirely exempt from that sensual brutality, which age has enabled my reason to
banish; thus I am not troubled with passions, and
my mind is calm, and free from all perturbations,

and doubtful apprehensions. Nor can the thought
of death find room in my mind, at least, not in any
way to disturb me. And all this has been brought
about, by God's mercy, through my careful habit of
living. How different from the life of most old men,
full of aches and pains, and forebodings, whilst mine
is a life of real pleasure, and I seem to spend my
days in a perpetual round of amusements, as I shall
presently show.

And first, I am of service to my country, and what
a joy is this. I find infinite delight in being engaged in various improvements, in connection with
the important estuary or harbor of this city, and
fortifications; and although this Venice, this Queen
of the Sea, is very beautiful, yet I have devised means
by which it may be made still more beautiful, and
more wealthy, for I have shown in what way she may
abound with provisions, by improving large tracts of
land, and bringing marshes and barren sand under
cultivation. Then again, I have another great joy
always present before me. Some time since, I lost a
great part of my income, by which my grandchildren
would be great losers. But I, by mere force of
thought, have found a true and infallible method of
repairing such loss more than double, by a judicious
use of that most commendable of arts, agriculture.
Another great comfort to me is to think that my

treatise on temperance is really useful, as many assure me by word of mouth, and others by letter,
where they say, that, under God they are indebted
to me for their life. I have also much joy in being
able to write, and am thus of service to myself and
others; and the satisfaction I have in conversing with
men of ability and superior understanding is very
great, from whom I learn something fresh. Now,
what a comfort is this, that old as I am, I am able,
without fatigue of mind or body thus to be fully
engaged, and to study the most important, difficult,
and sublime subjects.

I must further add, that at this age, I appear to
enjoy two lives: one terrestrial, which in fact I possess, the other celestial, which I possess in thought;
and this thought is actual enjoyment, when founded
upon things we are sure to attain, and I, through
the infinite mercy and goodness of God, am sure of
eternal life. Thus, I enjoy the terrestrial life in
consequence of my sobriety and temperance, virtues
so agreeable to the Deity, and I enjoy, by the grace
of God, the celestial, which He makes me anticipate
in thought; a thought so lively, as to fix me entirely
on this subject, the fruition of which I hold to be
of the utmost certainty. And I further maintain,
that, dying in the manner I expect, is not really
death, but a passage of the soul from this earthly

life to a celestial, immortal, and infinitely perfect existence. Neither can it be otherwise; and this thought is so pleasing, so superlatively sublime, that it can no longer stoop to low and worldly objects, such as the death of this body, being entirely taken up with the happiness of living a celestial and divine life. Whence it is, that I enjoy two lives; and the thought of terminating this earthly life gives me no concern, for I know that I have a glorious and immortal life before me.

Now, is it possible, that any one should grow tired of so great a comfort and blessing as this which I enjoy, and which the majority of persons might attain, by leading the life I have led, an example which every one has it in his power to follow? for I am no saint, but a mere man, a servant of God, to whom so regular a life is extremely agreeable.

Now, there are men who embrace a spiritual and contemplative life, and this is holy and commendable, their chief employment being to celebrate the praises of God, and to teach men how to serve Him. Now, if while these men set themselves apart for this life, they would also betake themselves to sober and temperate living, how much more agreeable would they render themselves in the sight of God and men. What a much greater honor and ornament would they be to the world. They would likewise enjoy constant

health and happiness, would attain a great age, and
thus become eminently wise and useful; whereas, now,
they are mostly infirm, irritable, and dissatisfied, and
think that their various trials and ailments are sent
them by Almighty God, with a view of promoting
their salvation; that they may do penance·in this life
for their past errors. Now, I cannot help saying,
that in my opinion, they are greatly mistaken; for
I cannot believe that the Deity desires that man, his
favorite creature, should be infirm and melancholy,
but rather, that he should enjoy good health and be
happy. Man, however, brings sickness and disease
upon himself, by reason, either of his ignorance or
wilful self-indulgence. Now, if those who profess
to be our teachers in divine matters would also set
the example, and thus teach men how to preserve
their bodies in health, they would do much to make
the road to heaven easier: men need to be taught
that self-denial and strict temperance is the path
to health of body and health of mind, and those who
thus live see more clearly than others what their duty
is toward our Saviour Jesus Christ, who came down
upon earth to shed His precious blood, in order to
deliver us from the tyranny of the devil, such was
His immense goodness and lovingkindness to man.

Now, to make an end of this discourse, I say, that
since length of days abounds with so many favors

and blessings, and I, not by theory, but by blessed
experience can testify to it—indeed, I solemnly assure
all mankind that I really enjoy a great deal more
than I can mention, and that I have no other reason
for writing, but that of demonstrating the great
advantages, which arise from longevity, and such a
life as I have lived—I desire to convince men, that
they may be induced to observe these excellent rules
of constant temperance in eating and drinking, and
therefore, I never cease to raise my voice, crying out
to you, my friends, that your lives may be even as
mine.

The following mystical pictures are not related to this book.

They have been included for your enjoyment.

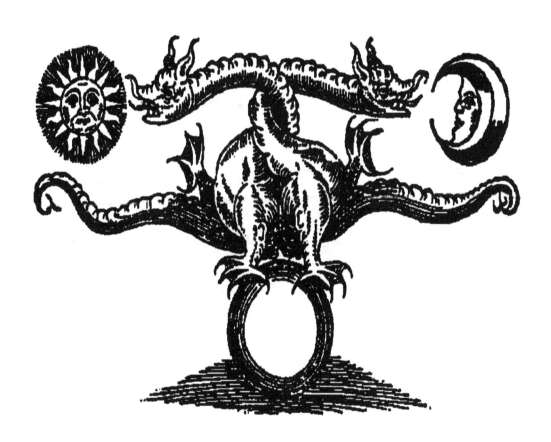

Pictures 1

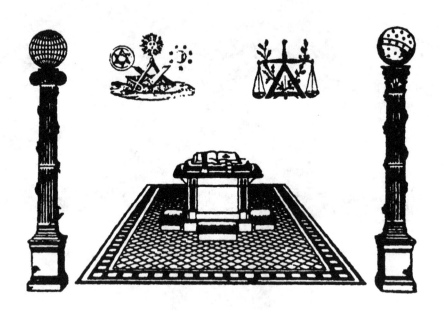

Pictures 2

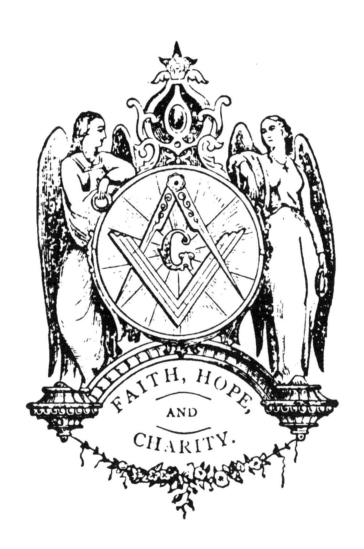

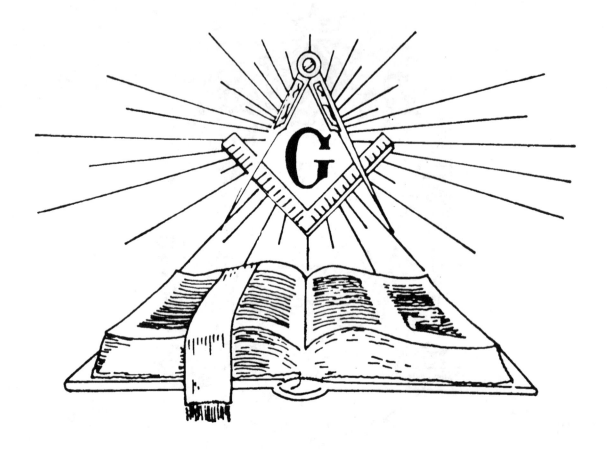

Pictures 4

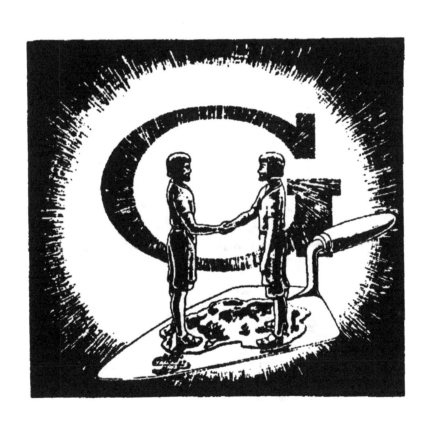

Pictures 5

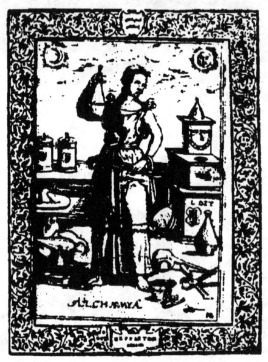

ALCHYMIA
(From Thurneyser's Quinta Essentia, 1570)

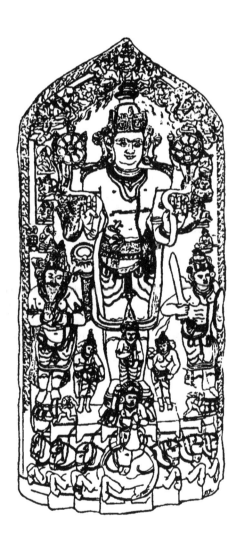

Pictures 7

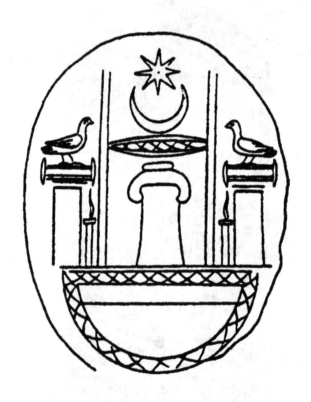

Pictures 8

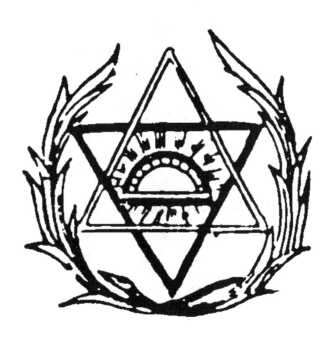

Pictures 9

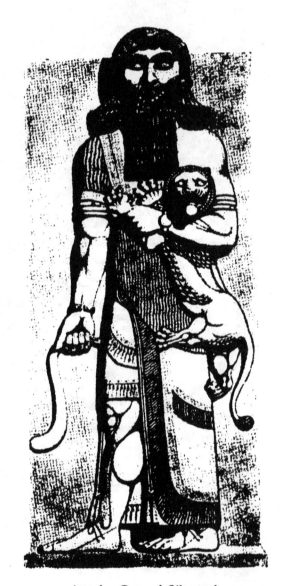

Assyrian Type of Gilgamesh

Pictures 10

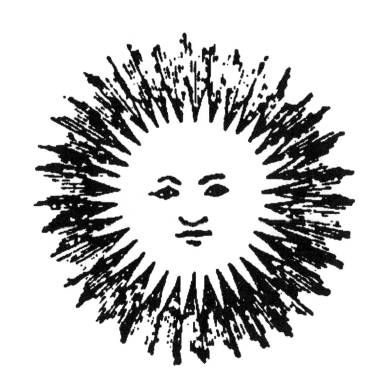

Pictures 11

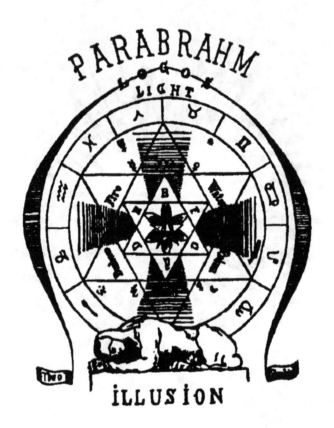

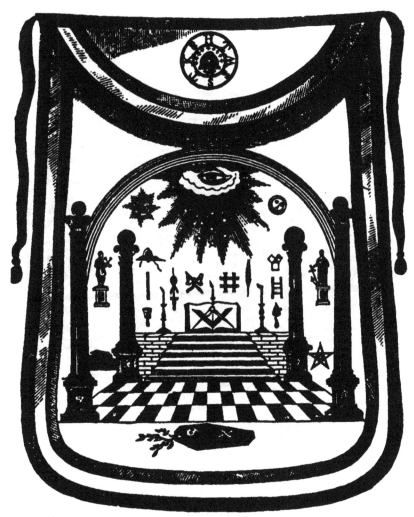

MASONIC APRON PRESENTED TO GEN. WASHINGTON
BY MADAME LAFAYETTE.

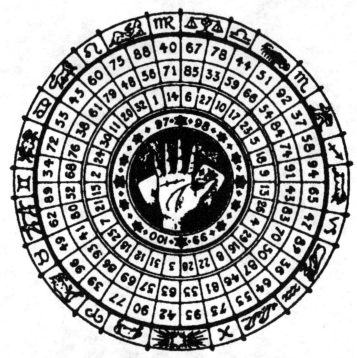

THE GOLDEN WHEEL

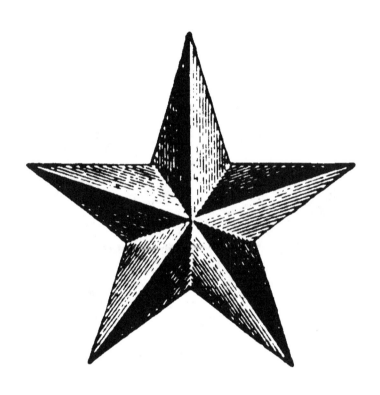

Pictures 15

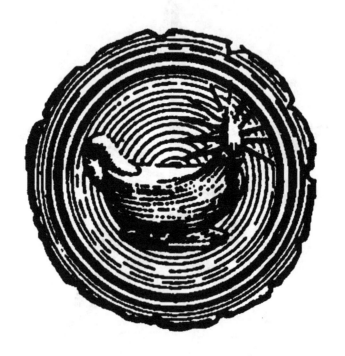

Pictures 16

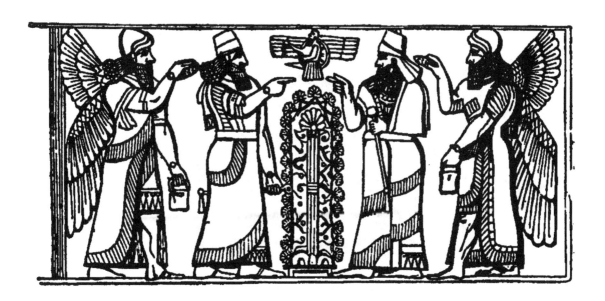

Pictures 17

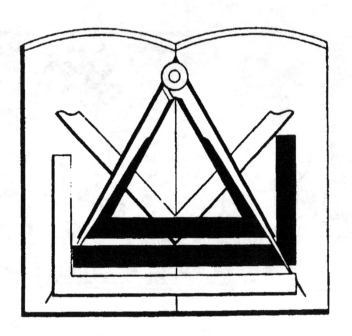

Pictures 18

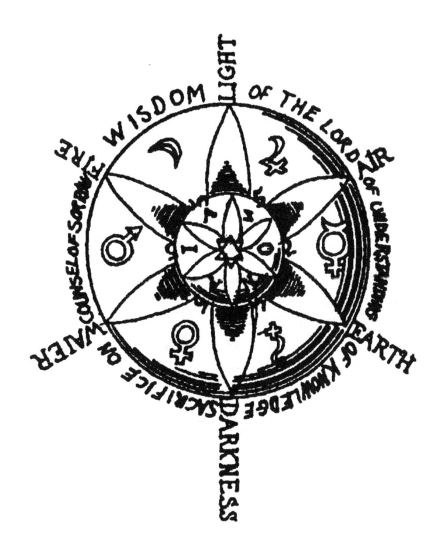

Pictures 19

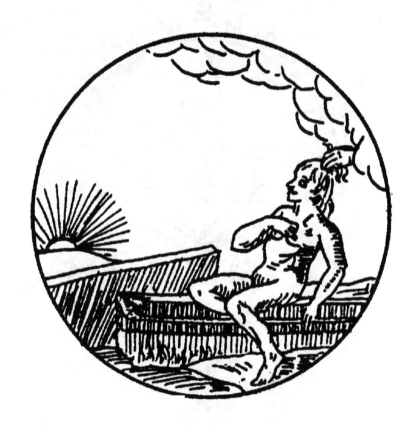

Pictures 20

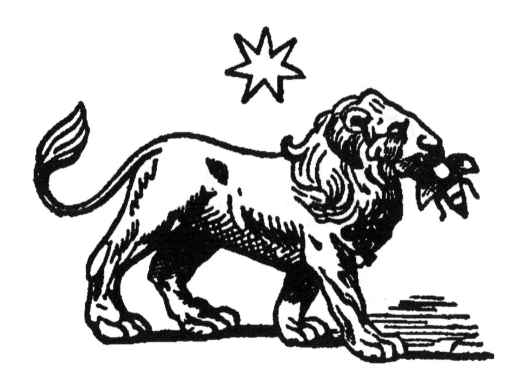

Pictures 21

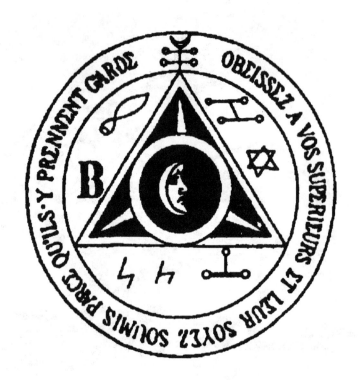

Pictures 22

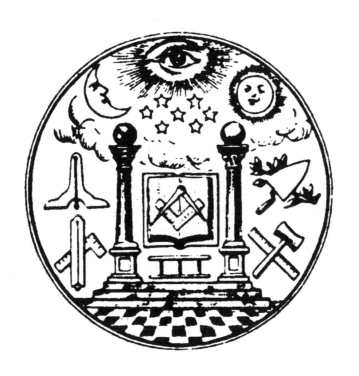

Pictures 23

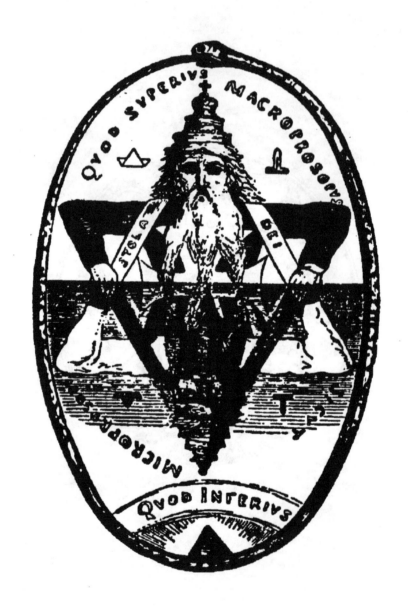

Pictures 24

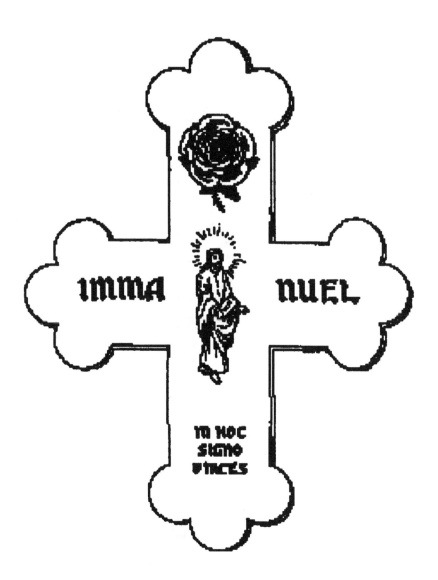

Pictures 25

MERCURIUS **DE** MERCURIO

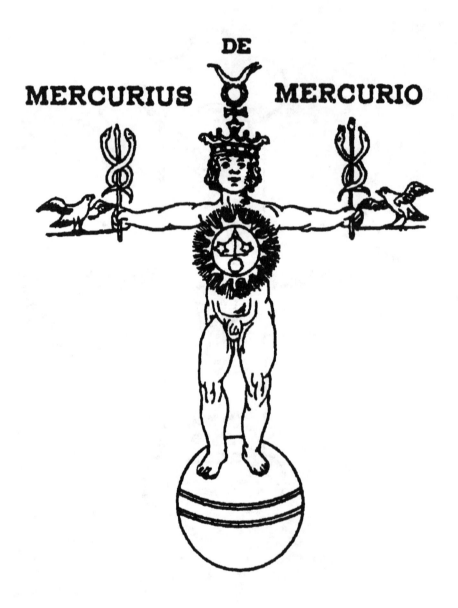

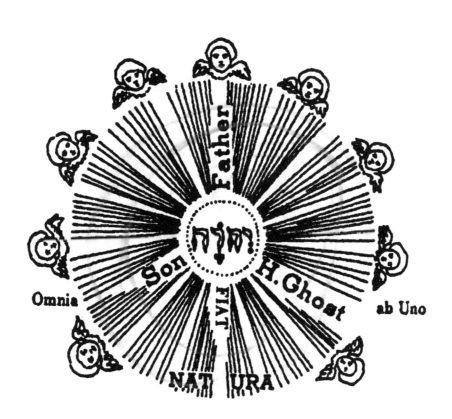

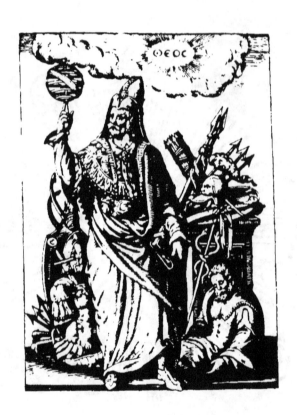

Pictures 28

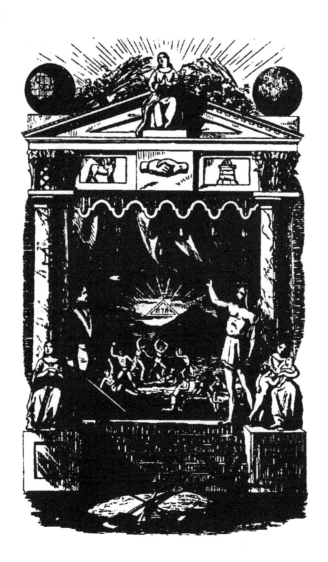

Pictures 29

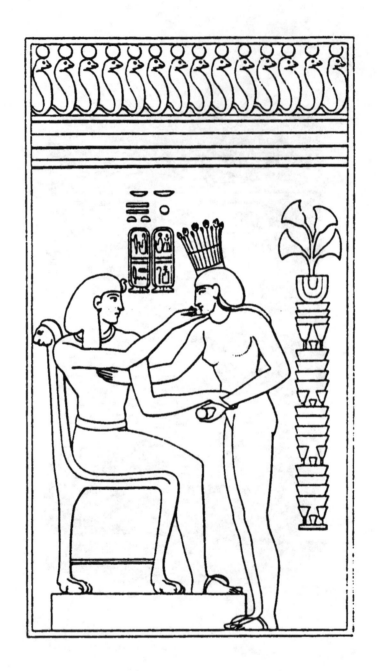

Pictures 30

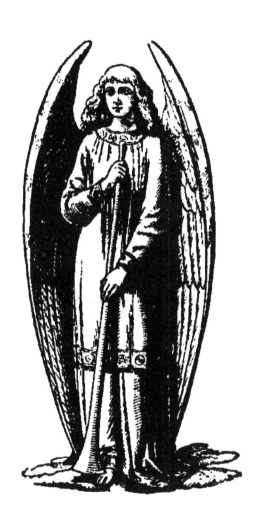

Pictures 31

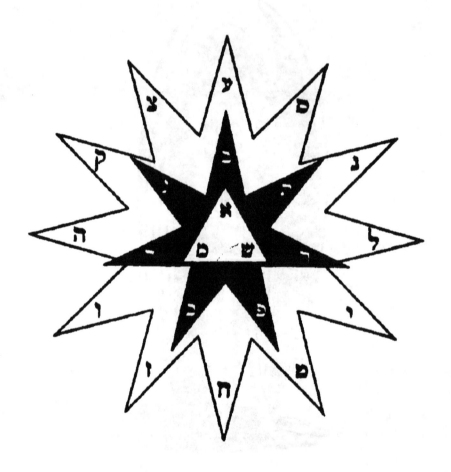

Pictures 32

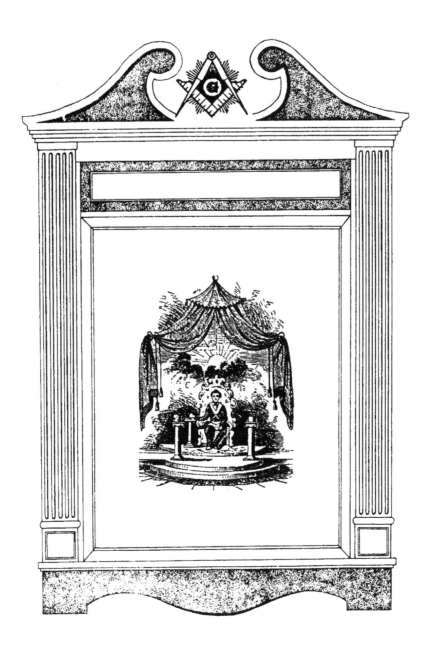

Pictures 33

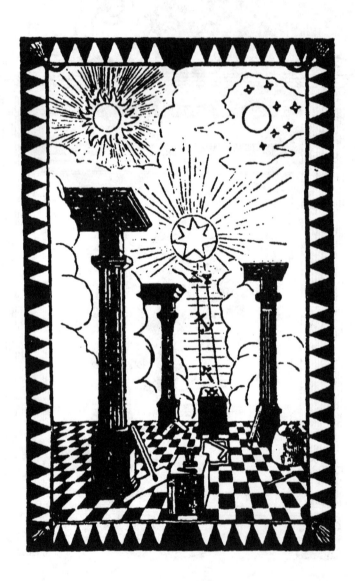

Pictures 34

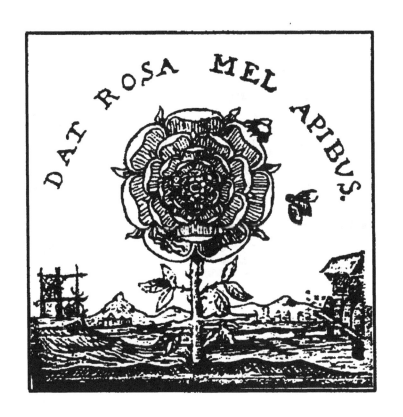

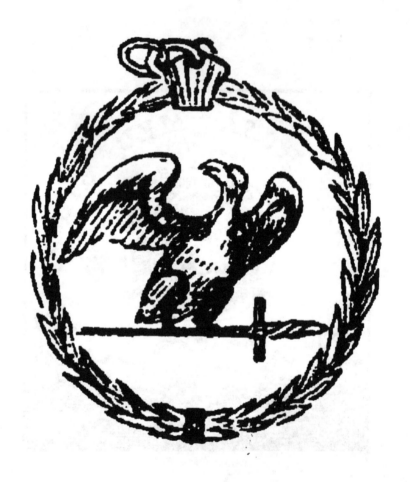

Pictures 36

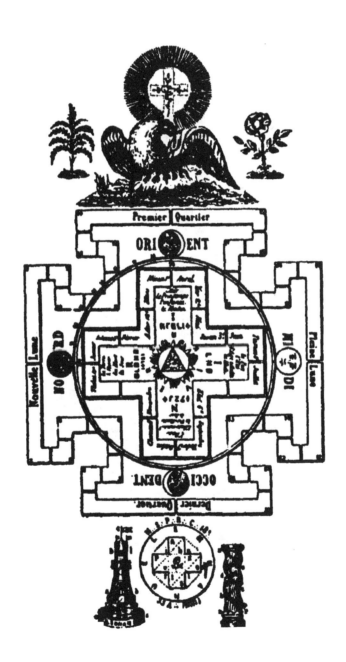

Pictures 37

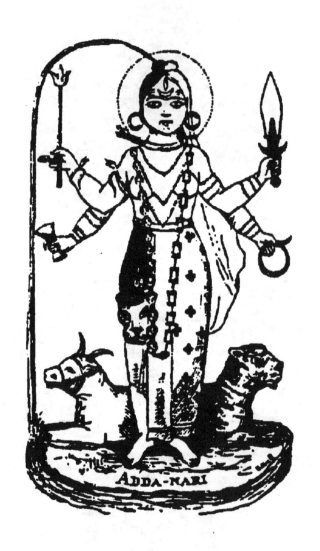

ADDA-NARI